Instructor's Guide to
Amput[...]
and
Prosthetics
A CASE STUDY APPROACH

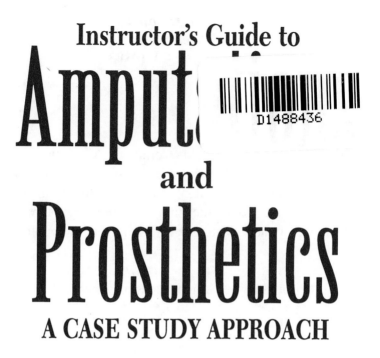

Bella J. May, EdD, PT, FAPTA
Professor, Department of Physical Therapy
Medical College of Georgia
Augusta, Georgia
President BJM Enterprise, PC

F. A. Davis Company ● Philadelphia, PA

F. A. Davis Company
1915 Arch Street
Philadelphia, PA 19103

Last digit indicates print number: 10 9 8 7 6 5 4 3 2 1

Printed in the United States of America

ISBN
0-8036-0084-4

F. A. Davis Company

CONTENTS

INTRODUCTION

Amputations and Prosthetics is designed to help students learn the basic concepts of the management of clients with amputations by working through typical case studies. This *Instructor's Guide* is designed to help you guide this learning process. You may choose to use the book as a supplement to the standard lecture format; the stimulus questions and activities may be used in the large class to generate discussion of the topic. You may also choose to use small study groups to work through each chapter and related activities, while using large group discussions for sharing information, answering questions, or exploring confusing or debatable points. The *Instructor's Guide* is meant to be a resource, particularly for faculty who may not have a strong background in the area of amputation and prosthetics. There are regional and facility variations in philosophy and approaches and variations in components. All of the materials in this manual have been used in class sessions with physical therapy and physical therapist assistant students.

One of the ways the textbook has been used is with a combination of small and large group activities. Students are divided into groups of 6. Each group works through the stimulus questions in each chapter as well as the more detailed items in this manual. Note that this manual is not designed to be used by students. Faculty circulate between the groups to clarify or guide the students to additional resources. It is not the purpose of the faculty to answer the questions for the students. Large group discussion sessions are scheduled following the small group activities. Each student group share their approach to the various questions with faculty raising points, asking students to justify their approaches or interventions and facilitating comparison of the similarities and differences between the clients. The instructor should schedule lectures to provide information beyond that offered in the text or for guest faculty, such as a prosthetist or vascular surgeon, who can offer special insights.

This *Instructor's Guide* also contains several suggested laboratory activities and a broad selection of test questions.

Additional resources

There are numerous resources on the Internet in the area of prosthetics. Northwestern University Rehabilitation Engineering and Prosthetic Orthotic Center (http://pele.repoc.nwu.edu/) provides information on current research projects and interesting brief videos in related areas. The Prosthetic Research Study (http://weber.u.washington.edu/~prs/) has information on the Washington Veterans Administration research program. The Orthotic and Prosthetic Network Connection (http://www.cloudnmet.com:80/~oandpnet/) includes web sites and listserves. All three have links to other sites.

CHAPTER 1

AMPUTATIONS AND PROSTHETICS: THEN AND NOW

Chapter 1 is designed to provide a historical overview of the field of prosthetics and surgery. Understanding the changes that have taken place over the years will help students appreciate current changes in prosthetic care and appliances.

Stimulus Questions

1. What do I bring to the client interaction? Place a mark on the visual analog scale to indicate your perceived level of competence in dealing with individuals with peripheral vascular disease.

I have absolutely no   I believe I could do idea
where to start   a competent job

What do you need to learn to change your position on the mark?

2. Review the historical developments presented in this Chapter. In study groups, discuss the changes that have occurred, impetus for the changes and become familiar with some of the terminology. Consider the future. What do you think are the important concepts to understand to be effective as a physical therapist or physical therapist assistant?

3. What seems to have been the major impetus for improvement in prosthetic components over the years? Why?

4. Discuss the role and function of the prosthetic clinic team. How does the physical therapists or physical therapist assistant fit into those functions?

5. If you have access to them, examine different prostheses to gain a better understanding of the effect of technological advances.

It is helpful to have prosthetic components readily available to supplement other audiovisual materials. Local prosthetists are usually quite willing to lend both current and older components. Local hospitals sometimes have old limbs in a closet. Students can be encouraged to feel the weight of older and current prosthesis, feel the softness of the cosmetic cover of endoskeletal limbs, and see the variations in socket configuration, among other comparisons.

CHAPTER 2

PERIPHERAL VASCULAR DISEASES

Chapter 2 provides an overview of peripheral vascular diseases, the major cause of amputations among the elderly. Depending on the program's curriculum, your students may have already studied this area or may be studying it concurrently. The chapter is not meant to substitute for a thorough study of the pathophysiology of vascular diseases.

Stimulus Questions

1. How would you diagnostically classify each of these people's condition? How would you differentiate between arterial and venous disease and between acute and chronic vascular disease? How prevalent are these particular diseases or syndrome? (e.g. how often do they happen, how likely are you to see this type of problem?) Can you describe each disease/syndrome from a pathophysiological point of reference?

2. Describe the pathophysiology of each diagnosis, differentiating among major signs and symptoms.
   What additional information do you need before you can evaluate or treat each client? Supplement the information in this chapter with any pathophysiology reference.
   Can you differentiate between the major signs and symptoms of each disease/syndrome? Can you identify the critical cues in each situation? What is the prognosis for life? for limb viability?
   How might the disease affect the lifestyle of each person (right now and in the future)?

What medication do you think each person would be taking? What do you need to know about the effects of these drugs?

3. What are the major medical and surgical strategies used in the management of these diseases?
   How much do you need to know about the medical and surgical treatment of each disease? Specifically, what do you need to know about a popliteal-femoral bypass to properly treat Mr. Pearl?
   What will be the effects of surgery on the respiratory system? What are some other types of vascular reconstructive surgery?

4. Physical therapy students: For each person, can you determine your course of action at this time?
   What data are needed to complete an evaluation? How would you prioritize the data? That is, given a limited time, which data do you need to obtain early and which can be delayed for later?
   What are the best sources of each datum (e.g., direct assessment, the medical chart) Explain your reasoning.

5. Compare and contrast the three people presented in the cases with the following two people:

   > Martin Greenberg, a 56 -year-old male, woke up this morning with severe throbbing pain in his left calf; it has gotten worse in the last hour. What would you suspect? How would you differentiate this from other acute vascular problems? What is the best course of action when you suspect a vascular emergency?

   > Barbara Matthews is a 61-year-old female who had a left total hip replacement 4 days ago and has been receiving PT for the last 3 days. Today,

when she is brought down to physical therapy, she complains of severe pain in her left calf.

Case Study Discussions

Diana Magnolia

This is a fairly typical client with a diabetic ulcer who may receive treatment as part of a wound care program. Some of the key points to consider include the effects of her work and lifestyle on her ulcer and how those effects might be moderated realistically. Her case represents a good focus for the disease itself and its similarities and differences with arteriosclerosis without diabetes. Emphasis can be placed on the effects of loss of sensation and ankle function on the ulcer. Discussion of client education and prevention programs is also appropriate.

Benny Pearl

You can use consideration of this case to focus on issues of surgical interventions, postsurgical precautions, and healing times. Using an atlas of vascular surgery to display pictures of the surgical procedure helps students visualize the process. Surgical techniques change over time and may vary with local preferences. It would be helpful to discuss the major types of surgical interventions with the students with some emphasis on local options. A vascular surgeon who has worked with physical therapy can be a valuable resource.

Charley Johnson

Chronic venous insufficiency (CVI) is not a cause of amputation. Many individuals with CVI may not receive any physical therapy. However, many individuals with arterial disease also have CVI, and consideration of this client's case helps students learn about CVI. It is important for students to understand the devastating effects of chronic edema on tissues. Edema limits the range of motion of the ankle, causes pain (which further limits mobility), and can damage subcutaneous tissue. Students need to learn how to evaluate and manage edema, since it is a continuous problem in prosthetic management.

Barbara Mathews
Martin Greenberg

These two cases provide a contrast between chronic and acute vascular problems. They can be used to help students learn how to handle acute vascular problems and differentiate symptoms between acute and chronic. A good lesson can be made around the types of pain associated with different diseases. Figure 2-1 illustrates the symptomatic differences.

CHAPTER 3

THE DIABETIC FOOT

Understanding basic concepts of the management of the diabetic foot is important. Even after the amputation of one extremity, preventive care is necessary, and the student must be able to identify the elements of preventive care and communicate the principles of preventive care to the client. It is helpful to bring in examples of adapted shoes and inserts.

This chapter is designed as a resource to faculty and students who do not have a diabetic foot clinic or facility in their area.

CHAPTER 4

LOWER EXTREMITY AMPUTATION SURGERY

It is important to note that this chapter discusses amputation surgery from the perspective of the physical therapist, rather than that of the vascular surgeon. After finishing this chapter, students begin to use the new terminology in earnest and may question the difference between the terminology used in the book and the continued use of the old terminology in practice.

Stimulus Questions

1. How do I feel about working with someone without a limb?
   Have I ever seen or worked a client without a leg?
   Do I feel differently about young or old clients?
   How do I feel about seeing or handling a residual limb?

2. For each client, describe what the surgeon will do with the bone, blood vessels, nerves, muscle tissue, and skin.
   What is the effect of each surgical techniques on the shape and condition of the residual limb?
   Do I understand the similarities and differences in surgical techniques for different levels of amputation?
   How long will it take for the incision to heal and what effect will the healing time have on postsurgical treatment?

3. What might the emotional aspects of amputation surgery be on each client?

Case Study Discussion

Each of the case studies is prototypical and can be used to compare and contrast major surgical approaches. Students need to consider how the major parts of the limb are handled surgically and reflect on the effect from a physical therapy point of view. There are many new terms in this chapter, and some time may be necessary to ensure that students have a functional understanding of   the such mechanisms as neuroma formation, myodesis, myoplasty, and skin flaps.

It is helpful to students to be able to see a surgical procedure, but no modern movies or videos of amputation surgery are generally available. Such videos may be available locally in teaching hospitals with vascular surgery or orthopedic departments. Seeing pictures or slides of a variety of residual limbs also helps students gain a better understanding of the surgical procedures. A discussion of the orthopedist and vascular surgeon's approach to amputation surgery may also be useful.

CHAPTER 5

POSTSURGICAL MANAGEMENT
OF AMPUTATIONS

The postsurgical treatment program is the focus of this chapter. The clients described in the case studies typify the major postsurgical approaches; consideration of their situations leads naturally to discussion of the effects of age on postsurgical goals and treatment.

Students need to understand the importance of timing in implementation of different aspects of the postsurgical treatment program. For each client, students can outline the appropriate precautions and contraindications, keeping in mind the variation in healing potential for individuals with and without vascular disease.

It is important for students to learn the effects of edema on healing and the importance of edema control. Students often question why, if the immediate postsurgical technique is the most efficacious in edema control, it is not used universally. It is difficult for students to understand the difference in philosophical approaches to amputation surgery between the vascular and orthopedic surgeons.

Although the results of the initial evaluation are given in the text, it is worthwhile to have students discuss each item, determine why the item is important, and discuss what could affect whether the evaluation would or would not be done in real life. Students need to develop their own evaluation plans and need to cope with the real-world pressures of limited time and short hospital stays.

Stimulus Questions

1. What is the effect of amputation surgery on each client's functional status?

   What are the significant data at this point?

   What might be each client's subjective complaints? Compare and contrast the different methods of residual limb post operative care; identify the major advantages and disadvantages of each.

   Discuss how you expect each person to respond to the amputation.

2. What is my evaluation plan for each client?

   What are the critical data at this time? Are there items you would add or delete from the initial evaluations as described in the text?

   What are your long- and short-term goals for each client?

   Assume each client has been referred the day after surgery. Which evaluation activities could you do on the first visit and which would have to be delayed?

   Prognosticate: Do you believe any of these persons is a prosthetic candidate? Why or why not?

   What factors must the physical therapist or physical therapist consider before taking goniometric measurements or performing a manual muscle test?

3. For each client, what is the optimal treatment plan?

   What would your initial treatment program consist of?

   What is your rationale for the treatment?

   Which parts of the treatment program can be best performed by the physical therapist assistant?

   What complications could arise during treatment? What would you do in response to each complication?

   How would the treatment program change over the first 2 - 3 weeks?

4. What are the long-term plans? What services are available for each client following discharge from the hospital? What home program would you devise for each client?

Case Study Discussion

Diana Magnolia

The evaluation depicts an individual who is ready for a functional treatment program emphasizing ambulation and self care. Care will need to be taken initially that exercises do not compromise healing. Post operative edema will be a problem causing pain and possibly interfering with healing. The client will need to learn proper residual limb bandaging and be encouraged to rewrap regularly. A shrinker may be advisable after the sutures are removed but Ms Magnolia will be discharged from the hospital with the sutures in place.

It is important for Ms Magnolia to learn the importance of preventing both knee flexion and hip flexion contractures. Given her size, and problems with the other leg, it is unlikely that she will be able to ambulate on crutches, although a trial with crutches is always advisable. She should be able to get around her house fairly well with the walker but will probably use a wheelchair for much of the day. She will probably not be as active as she was prior to amputation and will need to learn to spend some time prone daily.

The home program needs to include prone hip extension as well as such activities as SLR and hip abduction. Theraband works well for all of these exercises. A referral to home health may be advisable and the situation provides an excellent opportunity for students to discuss coordinated care over the long term.

Comparing and contrasting the emotional reaction to amputation between each client will highlight that Ms Magnolia has had time to prepare for the amputation during the care of her ulcer. She may actually welcome the amputation if it frees her from pain and the limitations of the ulcer. Care of the other leg is important, and the home program needs to include active or resistive exercises of the nonamputated extremity, including range of ankle motion, particularly in dorsiflexion.

Ha Lee Davis

Mr. Davis presents as a typical traumatic amputation and provides an opportunity to compare younger and older clients on a number of dimensions. The post operative program needs to include consideration of the cast. It needs to be inspected daily to insure that there is not too much drainage or pain. Edema will not be a problem unless he is not fitted with another cast when the first is removed for suture removal. At some point he will need to learn residual limb bandaging or be fitted with a shrinker for times he does not have the prosthesis. He will be able to walk on crutches limited only by the arm injury. Residual limb exercises can be quad sets as well as hip extension and abduction.

Benny Pearl

Mr. Pearl is the typical sedentary client who is reluctant to do much for himself. He will respond slowly and challenges the therapist to involve him in the exercise program. He should be able to learn to transfer and walk a little with a walker depending on the condition of the other leg. His exercise program needs to stress hip extension as he will probably sit much of the time and be prone to develop hip flexion contractures. Exercises for the other leg are also indicated. Residual limb bandaging will be difficult; a shrinker will probably stay on better than the bandaging but cannot be applied safely until the sutures are removed.

Betty Childs

Betty presents some unique problems.   The cause of amputation provides opportunities for exploring problems of life threatening illnesses and the special needs of young adults. Limb salvage procedures can be discussed as well as the effects of chemotherapy and radiation therapy on human function. Betty will have to cope with both the loss of a limb and the prognosis of cancer. She will need to be monitored throughout the period of chemotherapy and radiation therapy. Her participation in an exercise program will be determined by the physiological effects of the treatment. She should become independent with crutches quite quickly and the main focus of the exercise program will be to maintain strength and range of motion in the residual limb until she is ready for fitting.

CHAPTER 6

PSYCHOSOCIAL ISSUES

The psychosocial aspects of amputation are very important for clients of all ages. The differences in reaction to amputation between people who lose a limb suddenly due to trauma and those who lose a limb after long term problems such as vascular disease or osteomyelitis is useful to explore. Differentiating between phantom sensation, which is normal, and phantom pain, which can be debilitating, is important. It is helpful to students to role play situations between client and therapist or assistant.

Stimulus Questions

1. Compare and contrast the possible emotional responses of Diana Magnolia and Benny Pearl as compared to Ha Lee Davis and Betty Childs. What similarities and differences would you expect and why?

2. What would you expect the major psychosocial and economical concerns to be for each of the clients?

3. In laboratory or group sessions, role play the initial and ongoing contact between the therapist/assistant and each client. Practice asking and answering critical questions.

4. How do you feel about working with a child with cancer? Do you believe she ought to know her diagnosis or not?

Case Study Discussions

Diana Magnolia

Ms Magnolia's major concerns will probably focus around her ability to return to her premorbid level of activity and her job. Finances may be an issue and she may need help exploring sources of payment for an artificial limb.

Ha Lee Davis

Mr. Davis presents an excellent opportunity to discuss body image, adjustment to the loss of a limb and psychosexual problems. It may be helpful for students to explore what Mr. Davis would say or not say early after surgery and what behaviors he might exhibit during therapy.

Benny Pearl

Mr. Pearl may be concerned with finances as well and could form the focus of exploration of different types of resources available for rehabilitation and limb replacement. Mr. Pearl and well as Ms Magnolia may be concerned about the unamputated leg and harbor fears of losing that leg as well. Such fears may remain unstated unless the therapist provides an opportunity for the client to express them.

Betty Childs

Betty raises many psychosocial issues both from the point of having cancer and a potentially limited life span, as well as the amputation. Betty will, of course, be concerned with the reaction of her peers, particularly boys, as well as her ability to return to her previous life style. The family will be coping with the threat inherent in the cancer, the trauma of the medical care as well as the amputation. They will need as much support as the child. Depending on the focus of the course, Betty provides opportunities for exploring how one interacts with a child with a cancer diagnosis as well as what to say to a client who knows or does not know her diagnosis.

CHAPTER 7

PROSTHETIC COMPONENTS

Bioengineering and the introduction of new plastics and other materials have led to the development of a plethora of components for all levels of amputation. This chapter is designed to provide an overview of components with emphasis on generic concepts of each replacement part. Understanding the function of each type of component will enable students to interact knowledgeably with prosthetist. They will need to learn the specific names of appliances that are used in their community. Students also need to understand that the prosthetist is the most knowledgeable person about the advantages and disadvantages of each component including cost. The client benefits when therapist and prosthetist work together in making fitting decisions.

Stimulus Questions

1. Discuss the functions of the major components in the transtibial, transfemoral, and disarticulation prostheses.

2. Reflect on the extent to that a person's lifestyle affects prosthetic replacement and selection of components.

3. Assuming that each of these individuals is being evaluated by a prosthetic clinic, what components would you recommend for each of them. Why?
   If someone is not a prosthetic candidate, what would you recommend at this point?

4. For each major type of component, describe the characteristics of the client for whom that component would be most advantageous.

What would be the major characteristics of someone for whom the component is contraindicated?

Case Study Discussions

Diana Magnolia

The major concerns in fitting Diana Magnolia are her weight, the dysvascularity of the other leg, and her anticipated level of activity. The condition of the other leg encourages early fitting and a return to bipedal ambulation. Ms. Magnolia was active prior to amputation and mobile during the post-surgical period, so she should be able to return to an active lifestyle.

The socket of choice is the PTB, probably suspended by a sleeve depending on the contours of the lower thigh. Heavy individuals, such as Ms Magnolia, often have conical thighs, which may mitigate against adequate suspension with a sleeve. In such an instance, a supracondylar cuff with waist belt may be necessary. The sleeve will distribute suspension pressures over a broader area, and the cuff might be too tight around the distal thigh. A lightweight dynamic response foot, such as the Seattle Light foot, would provide enough response for her level of walking. An endoskeletal prosthesis would be more cosmetic and suitable for her needs.

Ha Lee Davis

Mr. Davis is a young, active individual who may be involved in sports and will certainly make many demands on a prosthesis. He is thin and probably has a well contoured distal thigh which would allow fitting of a PTB/SCSP prosthesis. Sleeve suspension is an equally valid choice. A silicone suction socket is not recommended for the first prosthesis but may be a choice once the residual limb has matured and stabilized. Mr. Davis would probably be able to make full use of a strong dynamic response foot such as the Flex Foot or the Springlite foot.

Benny Pearl

Mr. Pearl is a questionable candidate for prosthetic replacement. Many individuals with his degree of disability, level of amputation, and low level of mobility during the postsurgical phase of treatment do not become successful prosthetic users. If he *is* to be fitted, the simplest and lightest prosthesis is indicated. If the residual limb is large and flabby, he might be more comfortable in an ischial containment socket suspended by a pelvic band. However, the quadrilateral socket might be easier to don. A slide friction stance control knee is indicated for stability, combined with either the SACH or possibly a single axis foot, which increases knee stability. He is not likely to be able to walk well enough to utilize the properties of a dynamic response foot.

Betty Childs

Radiation therapy can actually burn the skin, and if this modality is applied to the residual limb or pelvic area, it will preclude prosthetic fitting until the skin has healed. Chemotherapy frequently leads to weight loss and malaise but does not necessarily preclude prosthetic fitting. It is important to fit a young person as soon as possible, but weight changes will need to be considered in when to fit. Cosmesis, comfort, and consideration for growth are important in selecting prosthetic components for Betty Childs. She will probably be quite active and could benefit from the lateral stability of the ischial containment socket suspended by a Silesian bandage. Suction is again not recommended for a first prosthesis, particularly when rapid growth will probably require frequent socket changes. The constant friction knee will serve her needs well until she is full grown, when a hydraulic system can be considered. There is some controversy over when to use hydraulics with a young person. There are some who believe in using hydraulics early because the unit can be moved into a new prosthesis to reduce costs. Since she will be active, a dynamic response foot is indicated.

CHAPTER 8

LOWER EXTREMITY PROSTHETIC MANAGEMENT

The training program for an individual with a prosthesis will, to a great extent, determine the eventual functional outcome, particularly with elderly clients. It is true that physiologically young and motivated individuals can learn to use a prosthesis well with minimal training, but those individuals do not represent the majority of the population. Early balance training is the key to eventual function. If the individual cannot learn to bear weight on the prosthesis, he or she will never have a smooth, energy-efficient gait. It is critically important for students to internalize the importance of early balance training and the need to avoid the use of a walker in any aspect of training. The walker mitigates against the normal gait pattern and against the function built into the prosthetic foot. The walker should only be the support of last resort, when it is obvious that the individual will never be ambulatory without a walker or when limited weight bearing is required for some reason. If time and visits are limited by financial concerns, it is better to spend the time on balance and weight support activities and knee control with the transfemoral prosthesis than to have the client walk with a walker up and down the treatment area using an uneven gait limited by lack of weight bearing on the prosthesis.

Comfort is critical to learning to bear weight on the prosthesis. If the prosthesis is uncomfortable, the client is not likely to want to bear weight on it. The student must learn to differentiate between the discomfort of something new and the discomfort created by a specific prosthetic fault. Careful inspection of the residual limb before, during, and after training sessions is key to preventing abrasions or sores that may interfere with prosthetic wear. Understanding why a particular prosthetic problem can lead to a specific complaint comes with experience, but the foundation can be built by using the case studies and asking students "If the client complains of . . ., what is the most likely cause?" Rather than blindly memorizing problems and causes, the students will understand and remember better if they see the relationships involved. The same concept applies to learning to recognize gait deviations and their causes. There are commercially available films and video tapes of gait deviations, and computer programs are being developed.

Additional Resources

The Rehabilitation Institute of Chicago makes available a film on transfemoral gait deviations. Although the film was made in the 1950s and depicts outdated components, it shows major gait deviations still seen today with good commentary on causes and corrections. "Gait Deviations of the Above Knee Amputee" is available from Paul E. Prusakowski, B.S., CP at O&P Digital Technologies, Inc. 2603 NW 13 Street, Suite 255, Gainesville, FL 32609. A CD ROM on transfemoral gait deviations is available from the Prosthetic Research Study, VIP CD-ROM Order, 720 Broadway, Seattle, Washington, 98122. A videotape on transtibial gait deviations is available from the Department of Physical Therapy, Medical College of Georgia, Augusta, Georgia 30912. An interactive computer program on transfemoral and transtibial gait deviations may be available in the future from the Department of Physical Therapy of the Medical College of Georgia. Since availability changes over time and new materials are developed, you may find current resources by contacting some of the amputee organizations on the Internet.

Stimulus Questions

1. What do I need to know about the client's condition to make fitting recommendations?
   What are your beliefs about the value of prosthetic replacement, quality of life, and the rehabilitation potential of each client?
   What conditions have to exist for a client not to be a prosthetic candidate? What does the research literature reflect on long term prosthetic use?
   Reflect on the extent to which a person's lifestyle affects prosthetic replacement and selection of components. Reflect on the psychosocial issues with each of the people. Are there concerns of funding?

2. How do you train an individual with a transtibial amputation to use a prosthesis? What do you already know how to do and what do you need to learn?
   Are there critical and non critical parts of a gait training program?
   What parts of the training program could be done by a physical therapist assistant?

3. What are the training similarities and differences between all levels of amputation?

Case Study Discussions

Diana Magnolia

Ms Magnolia will most likely become a functional prosthetic wearer. She will probably be able to get around the house without external support but will probably need a cane for outside activities. She will need to protect her remaining foot with proper shoe wear. Some clients tend to buy shoes in larger than needed sizes in the belief that larger shoes offer more protection. It is important for the client to understand that the size of the prosthetic foot is determined by the shoe given to the prosthetist and the remaining foot needs to be well fitted. A shoe that is too large can create sores and abrasions as much as one that is too small. Her training program needs to emphasize proper sock adjustment since her residual limb will probably shrink fairly quickly.

Ha Lee Davis

Mr. Davis will progress through the training program quite fast. However, it will be necessary to spend some time on balance and weight shifting training to make sure he develops the most optimum gait. He will also need to learn about sock adjustments and how to change shoes without changing alignment. Changes in heel height may be a problem when Mr. Davis wears sports shoes, dress shoes, or boots. A lift can be placed in the heel of the sports shoe to raise the height, and some adjustment is made by the type of foot, but major changes in heel height cause changes in alignment and can affect pressure on the residual limb as well as gait. It is an issue he will have to discuss with the prosthetist.

Benny Pearl

Mr. Pearl will be a training challenge. Learning to control the knee and to bear weight on the prosthesis will be critical. He will need to spend a great deal of time in the parallel bars until he is walking well enough to go outside the bars. Ideally, it would be beneficial if he could learn to walk with a quad or single point cane and it should be tried. It will be tempting to put him on a walker right away, but that choice should only be a last resort. He has the potential to become independent in ambulation in his home and for limited distances. He will probably continue to use the wheelchair for much of his mobility activities.

Betty Childs

Children learn to adapt to a prosthesis fairly easily. Once she masters weight shifting and knee control, Betty will be able to walk quite functionally. It is not likely that Betty will require support from outside the family; but, she is old enough to learn how to care for the prosthesis and will require that training. The family will also need to learn about sock use, heel height in shoes, and care of the limb. Changes in heel height will likely be even more of an issue with her, as she will probably wear sports shoes with low heels some of the time and more dressy shoes with heel some of the time. Her situation is similar to Mr. Davis', and it will be necessary for the therapist to discuss with the prosthetist the type of foot to be preferred.

CHAPTER 9

LONG-TERM CARE

Advanced training can take more or less time depending on the client's level of coordination, functional capabilities, and motivation. Students need to understand that it is important to review advanced activities with all clients because even active individuals do not always realize the scope of possibilities open to them. The list of organizations at the end of the chapter will be a useful resource for students as they enter practice.

Stimulus Questions

1. Discuss each of the client's possible long term psychosocial and financial adjustments to the loss of a limb.
   Compare Betty Childs and Ha Lee Davis in terms of adjustment to social and emotional life without a limb. What fears, concerns, and feelings will each have?
   Compare Diana Magnolia and Benny Pearl in terms of their adjustment to life without a limb. What might be their fears and concerns?

2. What problems might each person have to face to achieve full return to a meaningful life style?

3. What is each person likely to achieve functionally in the long term?

Case Study Discussions

Diana Magnolia

Ms Magnolia is likely to become fully independent and needs to learn activities such as stairs, ramps, carrying objects, and picking up objects from the floor. Because falls are a possibility, she should also learn how to minimize injury and how to get up from a fall. Her concerns will focus around financial issues: she may not be able to go back to work as a waitress because of the dysvascularity of the other leg. It may be that the amputated leg will be stronger than the remaining leg depending on the extent of the disease. She may eventually lose the other leg.

Ha Lee Davis

Mr. Davis may return to motorcycle riding and should be able to participate in all types of recreational activities. The loss of the leg should not prevent him from participating in any vocational areas. His major concerns will probably focus on his self image, his sexual being and his relations with women. Depending on his personality, he may have difficulty in his interactions with women or may use the loss of the leg to glamorize himself in the eyes of others. These, of course are extremes and he may well show little change in self image or acceptance.

Benny Pearl

Mr. Pearl will be more limited in functional outcomes than Mr. Davis. Mr. Pearl may be able to learn to go up and down steps–probably with a rail–but will most likely not reach the level of independence that Ms Magnolia will reach. The loss of the knee joint is a major difference between them and greatly affects functional potential. He is likely to continue to have problems with the other leg and may lose it as well.

Betty Childs

Betty is at the age where sexual interest, self image, and acceptance by others is important. Her concerns will focus on the effect of the loss of the limb on her acceptance by others, particularly boys but she will also be concerned about the cancer treatment, particularly if it is extended. Long term chemotherapy may cause fluctuation in weight and residual limb size that will necessitate close follow-up. Betty may benefit from involvement with a cancer support group for teens, and your students need to be aware of the available resources. Functionally, her abilities will be determined more by the cancer treatment than by the prosthesis.

CHAPTER 10

UPPER LIMB AMPUTATIONS

Although most individuals with an upper limb amputation are treated by occupational therapists, there are occasions when physical therapists and physical therapists assistants may need to work with such clients. The chapter has been written by a physical therapist from a physical therapist's point of view. The basic concepts of residual limb care apply equally to the upper limb, although shrinkage is not a major issue at this level. Since trauma is the major cause of amputation, the majority of clients are of working age. The lower the level of amputation, the more likely the individual will adapt to a prosthesis. The case study and discussion questions are contained within the chapter.

CHAPTER 11

THE CHILD WITH AN AMPUTATION

The child with a congenital amputation presents unique problems, particularly with the multiply limb-deficient child. The chapter is designed to provide an overview of the child with a limb deficiency and highlight the differences between adults and children. Students need to understand the importance of working with parents, because parents will carry out the majority of treatment activities and are critical in helping the child adjust to the disability. The chapter provides a brief overview of the technological aids available, particularly for the child with multiple deficiencies. More detail can be obtained with some of the references listed at the end of the chapter. There are also some videotapes that may be of value in this teaching session.

Stimulus Questions

1. Reflect on your feelings working with infant amputees and young children in general.

2. Classify Michael's amputations using appropriate terminology.
    Compare and contrast acquired vs. congenital amputations.

3. What do you need to know about normal upper limb growth and psychomotor development to plan and implement an ongoing treatment program for Michael for the next several months?
    What gross motor skills is the absence of his limb going to affect?

4. Develop a preclinic evaluation plan for each child.

   What critical data are needed to plan appropriate prosthetic rehabilitation?

5. Would you fit each of these children? Why or why not? If yes, what components would you select?

6. Compare and contrast the prosthetic rehabilitation program for each child.

Case Study Discussions

Michael Donnagin

Michael is ready for prosthetic fitting, probably with a preflexed one piece socket with a padded passive mitt. At 6 months of age, he is beginning to sit and will soon start bilateral activities. He needs something to oppose. The therapist/assistant must be able to teach the parents how to take care of the prosthesis, to explain the probable course of events over the years, and, most importantly, to help them understand that Michael has the normal needs of any child. The parents may need professional counseling, but the therapist can answer many questions about the habilitation process. Michael is most likely normal in all areas of development; play is the best therapeutic activity. Adjustment and acceptance of the prosthesis is easy in the infant. Problems may occur later as he starts interacting with other children. His adjustment will, to a great extent, be determined by the parent's attitudes.

Jenny Smith

Jenny can be fitted as soon as the residual limb is well healed. Some shrinking may be desirable if there is a significant amount of edema, but children grow fast and early fitting is advisable. At her age she will probably do well with an ischial containment socket with Silesian bandage, constant friction knee, and a dynamic response foot. Depending on her size, the range of components may be limited. Gait training will be relatively easy, and she should make a good adjustment to the prosthesis. As Jenny enters her teens, she may have some of the problems discussed earlier with Betty Childs. Again, it is vital that the parent are involved in all aspects of the rehabilitation program.

Mario Jonas

The decision to amputate the foot and fit Mario with an adapted prosthesis will be influenced by the potential for follow up in the clinic. The child may be fitted with an adapted PFFD prosthesis, which enables keeping the foot until he has grown enough to be able to create a reasonable residual limb. If an amputation is done, the type of prosthesis will be determined by the length of the remaining segment and the location of the knee center in comparison with the other leg. As Mario grows and the knee center rises, he will need to be fitted with a transfemoral prosthesis, probably similar to one for a knee disarticulation.

LABORATORY EXERCISES

The suggested laboratory exercises that follow were designed for a course that includes the study of peripheral vascular diseases. These are the handouts usually given to students as a guide to the laboratory activities. During the PVD clinical labs, intermittent compression machines, compression stocking measuring kits, and an ultrasound Doppler unit are available for student use. During the preprosthetic labs, transtibial and transfemoral models are available for the practice of residual limb wrapping.

CLINICAL SKILLS LAB #1:

PERIPHERAL VASCULAR DISEASE ASSESSMENT

This lab is designed to give you the opportunity to practice the skills necessary to provide effective care of individuals with peripheral vascular disease. Practice these skills through role playing. Both client and therapist must play their part to make this work. This lab is designed to help you make the transition from the classroom to the clinic.

As you prepare for this lab, it is a good idea to ask yourself the following questions:

- **What do I bring to the client?**
  Have I ever evaluated a client with peripheral vascular disease?
  What clinical skills do I presently have?
  Do I feel that it is important to actually role play a client or therapist in lab?
  Do I know what a Doppler is?
  Have I used or seen a Doppler used?

- **What do I need to know that I don't already know?**
  Do PTs use Doppler?
  How to use a Doppler?
  Why is it used?
  What new evaluation skills do I now need to learn?

- **How do I assure quality care?**
  Can I select and carry out evaluation procedures appropriately?
  What will I do with information from the evaluation?
  What are my clinical limitations with the Doppler?

Activities

In all labs, each student should perform each activity on at least two different people. You should to select people of different sizes and gender to ensure the greatest learning opportunities. Treat your lab partner as an actual client in the manner of approach, positioning, draping, handling, etc.

Evaluation Procedures

By the end of this lab, you should have applied each of these procedures appropriately.
- Doppler
  Become familiar with the instrument. Listen to venous sounds. Locate a venous valve. Listen to arterial sounds. Develop a scenario in which you as a PT may come in contact with a Doppler.
- Ulcer measurement and description
- Circumferential limb measurements
- Sensation testing
- Observation and description of skin conditions
- Checking lower extremity pulses
- Checking for rubor and pallor of a lower extremity
- Ankle/brachial index (ABI)

- Walking test for intermittent claudication
- Taking a history: asking relevant questions.

Diana Magnolia

1. With a skin pencil or face paint materials, draw the ulcer on the foot in the right place.

2. Choose and apply the appropriate evaluation procedures for this person. Record your findings in your notebook.

3. Identify specifically what other evaluative procedures, that you have previously learned, you would use in this situation. List those in your notebook.

Charley Johnson

1. Choose and apply the appropriate evaluation procedures for this person. Record your findings in your notebook

2. Identify specifically what other evaluative procedures, that you have previously learned, you would use in this situation. List those in your notebook.

Benny Pearl

1. Choose and apply the appropriate evaluation procedures for this person. Record your findings in your notebook Identify specifically what other evaluative procedures, that you have previously learned, you would use in this situation. List those in your notebook.

2. Identify specifically what other evaluative procedures, that you have previously learned, you would use in this situation. List those in your notebook.

CLINICAL SKILLS LAB #2:

PERIPHERAL VASCULAR DISEASE MANAGEMENT

This lab is designed to give you the opportunity to practice the skills necessary to provide effective care of individuals with PVD. One good way to practice these skills is through role playing. Both the client and therapist must play their part to make this work. This lab is designed to help you make the transition from the classroom to the clinic.

As you prepare for this lab, it is a good idea to ask yourself the following questions:

- **What do I bring to the client?**
  Have I ever measured a client for a pressure garment?
  Have I taken circumferential measurements?
  Can I adapt exercises I know to the problems of individuals with PVD?

- **What do I need to know that I don't already know?**
  Do I know the anatomical landmarks?
  Do I know the pathophysiology
  Can the client afford a pressure garment?
  Do I need a physicians order to fit a client with a garment?
  What are the manufactures guidelines for fitting a pressure garment?
  What is the proper technique for wrapping an edematous limb?
  What exercises will help clients with venous diseases? arterial diseases?

- **How can I ensure quality care?**
  What is the potential for doing harm; how can I avoid it?
  Are there other treatment choices?
  How is treatment recorded?
  How do I instruct the client?

Activities

In all labs, each student should perform each activity on at least two different people. It is important to select people of different sizes and gender for greatest learning opportunities. Remember to treat your lab partner as an actual client in the manner of approach, positioning, draping, handling, etc.

At the end of this lab, each student should be proficient in:

- Applying intermittent compression to an upper and lower limb
- Measuring an individual for an upper or lower limb compression garment
- Designing and implementing exercises for individuals with all types of PVD.
- Designing and implementing a walking program.

Charley Johnson

1. Practice wrapping the client's leg with elastic bandages from toe to groin for edema control.

2. Teach the client how to properly position the lower extremities at home at night. Use proper teaching techniques to improve the chances of compliance.

3. Apply intermittent compression to your lab partner's right leg.

4. Measure Mr. Johnson for a long leg pressure garment.

Clarice Anderson

Ms Anderson, 42 years old, underwent a right mastectomy 3 months ago. She is referred today because of persistent edema in the right upper extremity.

1. Practice wrapping the client's leg with elastic bandages from midpalm to axilla for edema control.

2. Teach the client how to properly position the upper extremity at home at night. Use proper teaching techniques to improve the chances of compliance.

3. Apply intermittent compression to your lab partner's left upper extremity.

4. Measure Ms Anderson for a long arm pressure garment.

Joel Jacobson

Mr. Jacobson is a 50-year-old business executive with chronic atherosclerosis and intermittent claudication.

1. Teach Mr. Johnson proper exercises to enhance the development of collateral circulation.

2. Teach and demonstrate proper walking techniques and plan a walking program to meet Mr. Johnson's lifestyle

INTERMITTENT COMPRESSION MACHINES

Intermittent compression equipment has been designed to reduce peripheral edema and venous stasis by stimulating the movement of lymphatic fluid from tissues to the venous system for elimination. Pressure is applied to the extremity through a pneumatic sleeve in a distal to proximal direction. Some machines provide a sequential series of pressures "milking" the fluid and encouraging venous return. Other machines provide all the pressure simultaneously, with the width of the sleeve exerting greater pressure on distal tissues. To be effective, the external pressure must be greater than the internal hydrostatic pressure in the tissues.

Intermittent compression machines come in a variety of sizes and complexity. There are small home models capable of providing straight intermittent compression to one extremity at a time. There are segmental units providing sequenced intermittent pressure and large, multiple-outlet machines, designed for use in the clinic or other facility, that allow for treatment of several clients or extremities at one time. The washable sleeves come in a variety of shapes and sizes and may be made of a clear polyurethane plastic or a blend of nylon and neoprene.

Indications/Contraindications

Intermittent compression is indicated for most clients by the presence of peripheral edema or lymphedema from such causes as chronic venous insufficiency, postphlebitis syndrome, postoperative or traumatic edema, or lymphedema from any cause. Skin ulcers or open wounds are not in themselves a contraindication to treatment and may actually be an indication.

Intermittent compression is *not* indicated in the presence of a thrombus or emboli or if one is suspected. Care must be taken in the use of intermittent compression in the presence of severe cardiac dysfunction, particularly left side cardiac failure.

Application

There are three variables that must be considered in the application of intermittent compression: the amount of pressure; the on/off cycle duration; and the length of treatment.

Amount of pressure: Pressure is indicated in millimeters of mercury (mmHg) and is generally determined by the client's systolic blood pressure. Manufacturers generally recommend an initial setting around 60 mmHg but no more than 20 mmHg below the client's resting systolic pressure. This is an acceptable setting for clients with edema not related to venous or arterial disease. For clients with venous disease, McCollough recommends a setting about 20 mmHg below diastolic pressure; he stated that in a recent study they found settings of 40-50 mmHg given for 1 hour twice a week to be effective in healing venous ulcers. The lower pressure will not place undue stress on an already compromised venous system and will not interfere with arterial flow.

On/off cycle: Research has indicated that an intermittent pattern of pressure is more effective than continuous pressure but there is little hard data indicating which cycle is most effective. Generally a 3:1 on/off ratio is used with the on cycle running 3 times the duration of the off cycle.

Duration of treatment: Once again research does not provide very specific guidelines. The severity and enduration will influence length of treatment to some extent. Generally, treatment should be at least for one hour three times a week and treatment of 2 or more hours is quite common. In a home program, the client may be encouraged to undergo treatment of one hour at least twice a day. Twenty or thirty minute treatments may be effective when using intermittent compression to reduce temporary residual limb edema preventing an amputee from donning a prosthesis.

Procedures: The following guidelines need to be considered in the application of intermittent compression.

1. Teach Mr. Johnson proper exercises to enhance the development of collateral circulation.

2. The client needs to be in a comfortable and relaxed position for a long-term treatment.

3. The limb generally needs to be positioned above heart level.

4. Sleeve cleanliness is enhanced if the limb is wrapped in a stockinet or, if there is an open wound, a plastic bag prior to sleeve application.

5. Wrinkles in stockinet, bandages or other wraps will indent on the client's skin.

6. Pressure is adjusted only during the "on" cycle.

Treatment effectiveness is greatly influenced by the maintenance of decreased limb volume through the application of a rigid dressing (Unna paste boot), pressure stocking or elastic wrap.

Bibliography

Ellingham C: Mechanical agents: external compression. In Sculy R and Barnes ML: Physical Therapy. Philadelphia, JB Lippincott, 1989

McCulloch JM: Intermittent compression for the treatment of a chronic stasis ulceration. Phys Ther 61:1452-1453, 1981

McCulloch JM, Hovde J: Treatment of wounds due to vascular problems. In Kloth LC, McCulloch JM, Feedar JA., Wound Healing: Alternatives in Management. Philadelphia, FA Davis, 1990.

CLINICAL SKILLS LAB #3:

POSTSURGICAL MANAGEMENT

This lab is designed to give you the opportunity to practice the skills necessary to provide effective care of individuals with amputations. It is helpful to practice these skills through role playing. Both the client and therapist must play their part to make this work. This lab is designed to help students make the transition from the classroom to the clinic.

Residual limb models are very beneficial for students to learn residual limb bandaging. A good resource is Lower Stump Bandaging Simulators" (above-knee and below-knee), product #LF-1064 from NASCO, 901 Janesville Avenue, Fort Atkinson, WI, 53538. Ph: 1-800-558-9595.

As the students prepare for this lab, encourage each to ask himself or herself the following questions:

- **What do I bring to the client?**
  Have I ever taught residual limb bandaging to an amputee?
  Have I ever instructed an amputee how to perform a preprosthetic exercise program.

- **What do I need to know?**
  About the surgery?
  About the client's mental status?
  About the client's general physiological status?
  What are specific evaluative and treatment procedures?

- **How can I ensure quality care?**
  What is the potential for doing harm and how can I avoid it?
  Are there other treatment choices?
  How is treatment recorded?
  How do I instruct the client?

Activities

In all labs, each student should perform each activity on at least two different people. Encourage the participants to select people of different sizes and sex for greatest learning opportunities. Instruct the students to treat their lab partner as an actual client in the manner of approach, positioning, draping, handling, etc.

At the end of this lab (two sessions), each student should be proficient in:

- Selecting and applying appropriate preprosthetic (post-amputation) evaluation procedures.

- Teaching an individual following an amputation proper bed positioning.

- Designing and applying selected pre-prosthetic exercises.

- Teaching and doing residual limb bandaging.

- Selecting and teaching appropriate methods of mobility.

- Teaching a home exercise program to a client and significant other.

Diana Magnolia and Benny Pearl are the clients for these labs.

1. Develop a preprosthetic exercise program for **each person** as follows:
   a. Exercise program you would institute in the first week after surgery
   b. Exercise program you would teach to the client and significant other on discharge 6 days after surgery.

2. Instruct **each client** on proper bed positioning.

3. Select the appropriate mobility activities for **each client**.

4. Teach residual limb bandaging to **each client** and **each client's significant other.**

5. Use the models to practice the appropriate type of lower extremity residual limb bandaging for **each client.**

CLINICAL SKILLS LAB #4:

PROSTHETIC TRAINING

This lab is designed to give students the opportunity to practice the skills necessary to provide effective care of individuals with amputations. Students should practice these skills through role playing. Both the client and therapist must play their part to make this work. This role playing is designed to help students make the transition from the classroom to the clinic.

The same format will be used for both the BK and AK gait labs. The first training lab will focus on the client with a transtibial amputation and the second on the client with a transfemoral amputation. Each group will prepare and present a role play of teaching selected activities to one of the clients. It is important that the role play be accurate and realistic. The role play will stimulate a class discussion on variations in training. The presentations should emphasize what would be the same and what would be different with each person.

Clients for the transtibial gait training lab are:

Diana Magnolia—fitted with a PTB socket with liner, supracondylar cuff, and waist belt and Seattle light foot.

Ha Lee Davis—fitted with a hard socket PTB/SCSP, and Flex Foot.

Clients for the transfemoral gait training lab are:

Benny Pearl—fitted with an ischial containment socket, pelvic band, Koleman stance control knee and SACH foot.

Betty Childs—fitted with a suction ischial containment socket with Silesian bandage, constant friction knee, Seattle foot.

Transtibial Gait Training Lab

Group A prepares the following:
> Closed environment activities: donning the prosthesis, static balance, and beginning mobility in the parallel bars with and without independent limb manipulation and intertrial variability.

Group B prepares the following:
> Gait training outside the bar with/without all types of ancillary support—but indicate which support is appropriate for each client. Closed environment activities with and without independent limb manipulation and intertrial variability.

Group C prepares the following:
> Getting up from and down on all types of chairs; getting up and down stairs and ramps; all complex closed environment activities; and care of the prosthesis.

Group D prepares the following
> Getting up from and down on the floor; kneeling; running (if appropriate); picking up objects from the floor; and all open environment activities with and without independent limb manipulation and intertrial variability.

Transfemoral Gait Training Lab:

Group B prepares the following:
> Closed environment activiteis: donning the prosthesis, static balance, and beginning mobility in the parallel bars with and without independent limb manipulation and intertrial variability.

Group C prepares the following:
> Gait training outside the bar with/without all types of ancillary supportóbut indicate which support is

appropriate for each client; and closed environment activities with and without independent limb manipulation and intertrial variability.

Group D prepares the following:

Getting up and down on all types of chairs; getting up and down stairs and ramps; all complex closed environment activities; and care of the prosthesis.

Group A prepares the following:

Getting up from and down to the floor; kneeling; running (if appropriate); picking up objects from the floor; and all open environment activities with and without independent limb manipulation and intertrial variability.

EXAMINATION QUESTIONS

There are many ways to evaluate attainment of competence. My belief is that the best approach to overall testing is a mixture of objective questions and essay questions based on simulated case studies.

The following represent a sample of possible objective examination questions. For each question, the correct answer is denoted by (x) after the distractor.

PERIPHERAL VASCULAR DISEASE

- Mr. Jones has been diagnosed as having a deep vein thrombosis. All of the following are potential complications *except*:
  - a. damage to the deep veins themselves.
  - b. a pulmonary embolus
  - c. a myocardial infarction (x)
  - d. inflammation of the veins.

- Ms Appleton has been diagnosed with chronic venous insufficiency and a noninfected venous ulcer. Your primary goal of treatment would be to promote healing of the ulcer through:
  - a. debridement, compression, and reduced weight bearing ambulation.
  - b. reduction of venous pooling by bed rest and exercises.
  - c. decreasing edema by compression, moderate elevation, and ankle pumps. (x)
  - d. stimulation of vascularization, prevention of recurrence, and limb protection.

- A rigid molded foot orthosis decreases pressure on bony foot prominences by:
  a. providing deep depression for bony prominences
  b. providing lateral stability of the foot
  c. supporting the forefoot during foot deceleration
  d. distributing the forces of weight bearing (x)

- Intermittent compression treatments would probably be beneficial for all of the following conditions *except*:
  a. chronic venous insufficiency
  b. chronic arterial insufficiency (x)
  c. lymphedema
  d. varicose veins

- Which of the following is *not* a classification of chronic arterial occlusive disease?
  a. Raynaud's phenomenon
  b. Thrombo angitis obliterans
  c. Arteriosclerosis obliterans
  d. Thoracic outlet syndrome (x)

- You note in your client's chart that comparative brachial and ankle blood pressures have been taken. Which of the following would be considered a normal reading?
  a. Ankle systolic pressure higher than brachial systolic pressure
  b. Ankle diastolic pressure higher than brachial diastolic pressure (x)
  c. Ankle diastolic pressure lower than brachial systolic pressure
  d. Ankle diastolic pressure lower than brachial diastolic pressure

- All of the following are appropriate treatments for clients with intermittent claudication *except*:
  a. moist heat with legs slightly elevated (x)
  b. elimination of all tobacco products
  c. medication enhancing vasodilation
  d. walk to discomfort, stop, walk again

- A client with chronic ASO is likely to exhibit all of the following symptoms *except:*
  a. pitting edema in lower leg (x)
  b. thickened toe nails
  c. no hair on lower leg
  d. thin, shiny skin

- All of the following are signs and symptoms of chronic venous insufficiency *except:*
  a. calf pain relieved by stopping walking (x)
  b. pain in both lower extremities
  c. pain relieved by sitting or lying down
  d. lower leg and ankle edema

- Mrs. Jones complains of sudden onset of throbbing pain in the right lower leg; the pain is not relieved by lying down. The right lower leg appears somewhat paler than the left lower leg. You would suspect:
  a. a popliteal artery embolus (x)
  b. vascular cramping elicited by exercise
  c. a deep vein saphenous thromboses
  d. chronic venous insufficiency

- Which of the following statements concerning arterial disease pain is *not* true?
  a. Elevation of the legs will relieve pain. (x)
  b. Pain is often described as cramping.

    c.   Rest or night pain can occur.

    d.   Pain occurs with exercise.

- All of the following statements about the characteristics of a venous ulcer are true *except:*
  a. Venous ulcers are often quite deep. (x)
  b. Venous ulcers often ooze a clear exudate.
  c. The area around a venous ulcer often shows hyperpigmentation.
  d. There is frequently edema associated with a venous ulcer.

- Ms Thorn, a 42-year-old nonsmoker, is being treated for a tibial fracture sustained in an automobile accident. During the course of conversation she indicates that she has difficulty handling cold objects. If she takes something from the freezer and has to carry it, her hands develop a stinging pain and turn pale. It is likely that Ms Thorn has:
  a. Raynaud's disease (x)
  b. Buerger's disease
  c. atherosclerosis
  d. arteriosclerosis

- Preventive foot care is especially important for individuals with diabetes since they are particularly vulnerable to foot problems. Which of the following is the *MOST LIKELY* mechanism leading to foot problems among individuals with diabetes?
  a. Diminished sensation and circulation lead to multiple foot fractures, which heal poorly.
  b. Diabetic neuropathies lead to imbalances in the muscles of the feet.

  c. Diminished sensation decreases the person's awareness of poorly fitting shoes. (x)

  d. Diabetic neuropathies leads to bone demineralization and changes in the autonomic nervous system.

Susan Sims has a superficial ulcer distally on the (R) leg just proximal to her medial malleolus. Answer the next three questions in relation to Ms. Sims.

- What other clinical symptoms do you expect her to have?

  a. Pain in the calf, paresthesia, pallor, and absence of pulses in the (R) LE

  b. Marked edema of the (R) LE and acute pain in (R) calf when (R) ankle is passively dorsiflexed

  c. Decreased pulses in the (R) LE and severe cramping pain in (R) calf when Susan walks

  d. Edema of (R) ankle and foot; brownish discoloration and watery exudate around the ulcer. (x)

- Which of the following is the most effective advice to give Ms. Sims?

  a. When sitting, keep both legs elevated on at least three pillows.

  b. When lying down, keep both knees bent over a pillow and do ankle pumps.

  c. When sitting, keep your legs up on a stool and do ankle pumps. (x)

  d. When lying down, keep the leg elevated no less than 45 or 50 degrees.

- Which of the following is the most accurate statement about exercises for Ms. Sims?

  a. Ambulate to tolerance several times a day.

  b. Perform active ankle exercises with feet level with heart. (x)

    c.   Use Theraband for resistive lower extremity exercises.

    d.   Exercises are contraindicated until the ulcer is healed.

Jack Palance, a 60-year-old business executive, comes to physical therapy with the referral: "Atherosclerosis - please evaluate and treat." Mr. Palance tells you that he cannot walk very far because of pain in his right calf, and that he is very busy and has little time for this problem. It is evident that he expects you to "fix" it. Answer the next three questions in relation to Mr. Palance.

- Which of the following would be the most accurate statement about Mr. Palance's calf pain?
  a.   It probably eases when he stops to rest or sit. (x)
  b.   It is probably better when he lies down than when he stands.
  c.   It would probably ease if he would keep walking and not give in to it.
  d.   It is probably directly related to his stress level.

- What other symptoms is Mr. Palance most likely to have?
  a. Pallor and paresthesia of the (R) foot, inability to move the (R) ankle, absence of pedal pulse
  b. Marked edema (R) LE and acute pain in the (R) calf when the (R) ankle is passively dorsiflexed
  c. Pitting edema of the (R) ankle and foot; brownish skin discoloration of both lower extremities
  d. Thick, opaque toenails; dry, flaky skin; ith little or no hair on both legs; diminished sensation (R) foot (x)

- Which of the following home activities would be most beneficial for Mr. Palance at this time?

    a. Put a heating pad on his (R) foot and ankle b.i.d.

    b. Soak (R) foot and ankle in water 105-110 degrees b.i.d.

    c. Walk to tolerance in his neighborhood daily. (x)

    d. Join a low impact aerobic class at the local YMCA.

- Which of the following is the most accurate description of rest pain in reference to patients with peripheral vascular disease?

  a. A heavy, aching pain in the lower extremities that comes on with elevation of the legs

  b. A sharp cramping pain in the calf that increases with foot dorsiflexion or manual squeezing

  c. A sharp stabbing pain that comes on in the morning when the patient first gets out of bed

  d. A cramping pain in the foot or calf that comes on during the night (x)

- Mr. Riddle is referred to you because of chronic TAO. Which of the following is the most accurate description of TAO?

  a. Affects mostly males aged over 60; affects the lower extremities; characterized by thrombolytic occlusion of medium and small vessels.

  b. Affects mostly males between 20-40 years of age; affects arteries and veins in lower and some upper extremities; characterized by thrombolytic occlusion of medium and small vessels. (x)

  c. Affects males and females usually over the age of 50; affects upper and lower extremities; characterized by the formation of arteriosclerotic plaques high in lipids.

  d. Affects mostly young females; affects upper with some lower extremity involvement; patients are cold sensitive; characterized by vasospasm of small arteries.

LOWER EXTREMITY AMPUTATION SURGERY

- All of the following statements regarding transtibial prosthetic surgery are true *except:*
  a. The muscles are divided and removed allowing for optimal healing.
  b. Dissection is carried down through the deep fascia to the bone.
  c. Nerves are severed high with a sharp scalpel and allowed to retract.
  d. Blood vessels are ligated or cauterized.

- Which of the following statements most accurately defines the term *myodesis:?*
  a. Suturing anterior and posterior compartment muscles together.
  b. Shaving and beveling posterior compartment muscles.
  c   Suturing anterior and posterior compartment muscles to the bone.
  d. Using the fishmouth shape to close the incision surgically.

- Which of the following statements is the most accurate reason for the use of the long posterior flap in transtibial amputation surgery for vascular disease?

  a. It provides a better weight-bearing surface for the residual limb .
  b. There is a lower probability of neuroma development.

   c.   There is better collateral circulation in the posterior flap.

   d.   It places the incision away from any bony prominence.

- Which of the following statements is the reason for most problems with the Symes amputation?
  a.   The amputee must wear his or her prosthesis to walk about the house.
  b.   Many prosthetic adjustments are required to maintain adequate fit.
  c.   There is continued intermittent claudication in the triceps surae muscles.
  d.   Faulty surgical technique can cause the heel flap to be misplaced. (x)

- Myodesis may be contraindicated in the dysvascular transtibial amputation procedure because:
  a.   the encircling sutures may cause constriction of local muscles (x)
  b.   the procedure alters the shape of the residual limb
  c.   the remaining length of tibia is not adequate for this procedure
  d.   myodesis is never performed with a transtibial amputation

- Which of the following is the most common way of managing the fibula in amputations through the middle third of the limb?
  a.   Cutting the fibula about 1 cm below the tibia
  b.   Excising the fibula totally
  c.   Sectioning the tibia and fibula the same length
  d.   Cutting the fibula about 1 cm above the tibia (x)

- Which of the following is *not* a cause of amputation wound healing failure?
  a. Post operative incisional infection
  b. Post operative residual limb edema
  c. Poorly controlled IDDM
  d. Poor residual limb muscle strength (x)

- Which of the following statements about the Chopart amputation is *not* true?
  a. The procedure is used frequently in the presence of dysvascularity. (x)
  b. The procedure allows end weight bearing on a normal heel pad.
  c. The amputated limb length is not affected by this procedure.
  d. The procedure is Indicated for a child with a fibular amelia.

- The Symes level is *the most* appropriate choice for all of the following conditions *except:*
  a. a teenager with a severe club foot deformity that did not respond to casting.
  b. a woman with a traumatic avulsion of the foot from an automobile accident.
  c. a client with a diabetic ulcer on the first metatarsal that does not heal. (x)
  d. a client with chronic osteomyelitis of the cuboid bones.

- An advantage of the hip disarticulation amputation over the hemipelvectomy is that:
  a. the ipsilateral ischial tuberosity remains, which makes sitting easier. (x)
  b. it is less painful

   c. for tumors of the proximal thigh, it provides a greater margin of normal tissue

   d. it is considered to be technically less difficult because fewer muscle masses are transected.

- Which of the followingstatements about the standard Symes amputation is *not* true?

   a. It provides an end weight bearing area in the residual limb.

   b. It is a disarticulation type of surgery.

   c. It preserves all normal muscle attachments.

   d. It does not require a prosthesis for functional ambulation.

Matching: Match the item in column A with the correct amputation level from Column B.

Column A

___ 2/3 of femur left
___ Ankle disarticulation
___ less than 5 cm of tibia
___ removal of sacroiliac joint
    and ilium
___ no bone is cut
___ 5cm below greater trochanter

Column B

A. Chopart
B. Short transtibial
C. Short transfemoral
D. Symes

E. Long transfemoral
F. Disarticulation
G. Transpelvic
H. Hip disarticulation

POSTSURGICAL MANAGEMENT OF AMPUTATIONS

- In the early postoperative period, use which of the following positions would advise a person with a transtibial amputation to use in bed?
  a. Supine: residual limb elevated on a pillow with the knee straight; sidelying: on the amputated side only with a pillow between the legs.
  b. Supine: Residual limb straight with hip and knee extended; sidelying: on the amputated side only without any pillow between the legs.
  c. Supine: residual limb elevated on a pillow with the knee flexed; sidelying: on the nonamputated side only without a pillow between the legs.
  d. Supine: residual limb straight with hip and knee extended; sidelying: on the nonamputated side only with a pillow between the legs. (x)

- Which of the following is *not* an appropriate short term goals for a patient who has just undergone a transtibial amputation for arteriosclerosis obliterans (ASO)?
  a. Promote independent mobility
  b. Increase strength weak muscles
  c. Prevent knee flexion contracture
  d. Increase residual limb circulation (x)

- You have received an outpatient referral for a person with a healed transtibial amputation and a flabby residual limb. The person is a questionable prosthetic candidate because of multiple physical problems. What would be the most appropriate course of action at this time?

a. Initiate a preprosthetic program of mobility training, exercises, and residual limb care, and see how the client responds. (x)

b. Call the physician and request a prescription for a temporary prosthesis to evaluate potential for prosthetic fitting.

c. Teach the client and family residual limb bandaging and send them home; reevaulate after 2 months.

d. Speak to the family in private and express your concerns about the client's poor potential for prosthetic rehabilitation. (x)

- Early in the postoperative period, you can best help an individual begin to adjust to the loss of a limb by doing which of the following?

    a. Ask the local prosthetists to bring some sample legs and components to the department for the client to see and handle.

    b. Provide detailed written and oral information about the prosthesis and the prosthetic rehabilitation program.

    c. Explain to the client that care of the other limb is critical to preserve the limb and the ambulation potential.

    d. Schedule the person for treatment when individuals with prostheses are in the department and walking. (x)

- All of the following statements about postamputation crutch training are true *except:*

    a. The amputee who cannot learn to walk on crutches will not be able to learn to use a prosthesis. (x)

b. Crutch walking is a good way for the amputee to learn new patterns of body balance and coordination.

c. Some dysvascular amputees do not have adequate circulation in the remaining extremity to tolerate the pressure of walking.

d. Many elderly amputees are afraid to try to walk with crutches on the one remaining extremity.

• Mrs Karen Apple, 82-year-old widow who lives alone in an apartment in a retirement community, has recently undergone a transtibial amputation for arteriosclerotic gangrene. You go to see her 2 days after surgery and she says she does not want any therapy and does not want to get out of bed; she requests that you just leave her alone. Which of the following is your best course of action?

a. Ask her how she feels about the amputation and what she would like to accomplish before discharge from the hospital. (x)

b. Tell her the doctor has ordered physical therapy and that she will feel better if she lets you give her exercises.

c. Leave her and report to the doctor you cannot treat a client who is not willing to be treated

d. Ignore her comments and begin the evaluation interview, asking if she's been out of bed yet and if she can sit up in bed by herself.

• Ms. Evans has been referred 24 hours after transtibial amputation. On entering the room, you find her lying in bed with a pillow under her right knee and her residual limb wrapped in a soft gauze dressing up to midthigh. After you greet her the *first* thing you want to do is:

   a.   remove the soft gauze dressing to inspect the incision.
   b.   remove the pillow from under her knee. (x)
   c.   have her come to sitting position at the side of the bed.
   d.   check the range of motion of her arms.

- Which of the following activities would probably be part of your *initial* treatment program with Ms. Evans?
  1. proper bed positioning
  2. crutch walking
  3. sitting over edge of bed
  4. gluteal setting
  5. resistive quad exercises of the residual limb
  6. general upper extremity strengthening

   a.   1, 3, 5
   b.   2, 3, 4, 6
   c.   1, 3, 4, 6 (x)
   d.   1, 4, 5

- A temporary prosthesis is valuable in the rehabilitation of the elderly individual with a transtibial (BK) amputation because it:
  a. eliminates phantom sensation.
  b. slows stump muscle atrophy.
  c. prevents hip flexion contractures.
  d. promotes continued ambulation. (x)

- Which of the following is the most common pattern of residual limb contractures following transtibial amputation?
  a. Hip in flexion, knee in extension.
  b. Hip in adduction and flexion, knee in flexion.

    c.   Hip in extension and abduction, knee in extension.
    d.   Hip in flexion, knee in flexion. (x)

- All of the following may be contributing factors to the failure of an amputation incision to heal *except:*
  a.   residual limb edema.
  b.   postoperative infection.
  c.   ligation and resection of major nerves. (x)
  d.   bleeding from the edges of the wound.

- For a client referred 4 days after transtibial amputation, which of the following would *not* be part of the initial data collection?
  a.   circumferential measurements of residual limb (x)
  b.   gross strength of the remaining lower limb
  c.   healing status and condition of the incision
  d.   client's ability to follow directions

- Which of the following is *not* an important part of the postamputation client education program?
  a.   Residual limb bandaging.
  b.   Care of the remaining lower extremity.
  c.   Selecting prosthetic components. (x)
  d.   Residual limb hygiene.

- You are treating a client who underwent a transtibial amputation for atherosclerotic gangrene yesterday. The client is alert and responsive. He has a soft gauze dressing around the residual limb and up to midthigh. All of the following would be appropriate activities to initiate today EXCEPT:
  a.   moderate residual limb wrapping over the gauze wrap

    b.   isometric exercises for the hip extensor muscles on the amputated side
    c.   resistive exercises to pain tolerance for the knee musculature on the amputated side. (x)
    d.   strengthening exercises for the upper extremities and remaining lower limb.

- All of the following are functions of residual limb wrapping *except*:
    a.   increasing collateral circulation. (x)
    b.   controlling postoperative edema.
    c.   reducing the circumferential dimensions
    d.   promoting incisional healing.

- For which of the following questions is an accurate answer most crucial on the day after amputation surgery?
    a.   Has the client ever walked with assistive devices?
    b.   Has the client ever had physical therapy?
    c.   Has the client been out of bed yet? (x)
    d.   Dose the client want to be fitted with a prosthesis?

- For the person resting in bed after transfemoral amputation, the optimal supine position is with the residual limb:
    a.   elevated on a pillow and slightly abducted.
    b.   flat on the bed and slightly abducted.
    c.   elevated for drainage and slightly adducted.
    d.   flat on the bed and slightly adducted. (x)

PROSTHETIC COMPONENTS

- In comparison with the PTB with a soft liner, the hard-socket PTB prosthesis provides all of the following *except*:
  a.   cushioning for sensitive skin. (x)
  b.   a more intimate fit.
  c.   good sensory feedback.
  d.   more ease in cleaning.

- Which of the following is *not* a method of suspending a transtibial prosthesis?
  a.   Thigh corset
  b.   Pelvic belt (x)
  c.   Medial condylar wedge
  d.   Supracondylar strap

- The major difference between the PTB and the PTS prosthesis is:
  a.   degree of socket flexion.
  b.   methods of suspension. (x)
  c.   areas of stabilization.
  d.   areas of weight bearing.

- The major benefit of the supracondylar cuff as a method of suspending the PTB prosthesis is that it:
  a.   allows full use of thigh muscles. (x)
  b.   provides medial/lateral knee stability.
  c.   stabilizes short limbs when heavy objects are lifted.
  d.   is highly cosmetic.

- The addition of a steel shank to the shoe of an individual with a transmetatarsal amputation may be necessary to:

a. prevent proximal distal irritation of the residual limb caused by premature drop-off during gait. (x)

b. prevent excessive pressure on the heel of the residual limb caused by premature heel strike on the short side.

c. support the anterior portion of the shoe on the amputated side during prosthetic swing phase of gait.

d. assure appropriate cosmesis by maintaining the shape of the shoe worn on the amputated side.

- Which of the following statements is *not* true concerning any prosthetic replacement of a limb (upper or lower extremity)?
  a. The prostheses must be as cosmetic as possible.
  b. The prostheses must be as functional as possible.
  c. The prostheses must be as light as possible.
  d. The prostheses must be as mechanically simple as possible. (x)

- Which of the following statements about the ischial containment socket is *not* true?
  a. The ischium is contained within the socket.
  b. The AP dimension is larger than the ML dimension.
  c. The client walks sitting on top of the posterior wall. (x)
  d The lateral wall cups over the greater trochanter.

- Which of the following best describes the major advantage of any hydraulic knee mechanism as compared to any mechanical knee joint?
  a. The hydraulic mechanism is cheaper and easier to maintain over the life of the limb.

b. The hydraulic mechanism varies swing phase control in response to amputee cadence. (x)

c. The hydraulic mechanism provides stance phase control at any point in the gait cycle.

d. The hydraulic mechanism is generally lighter thereby requiring less energy in gait.

- Which of the following is the best description of the type of prosthesis used for someone with a modified Symes amputation?

  a. Lateral opening PTB prosthesis with some weight bearing on the patellar tendon and some at the end of the stump.

  b. Closed expandable PTB prosthesis with weight bearing partially on the patellar tendon and partially at the end of the stump.

  c. Posterior opening prosthesis reaching to tibial tubercle with weight bearing at the end of stump.

  d. Leather laced prosthesis reaching to below the tibial tubercle with weight bearing at end of the stump.

- The PTBSCSP method of suspending the transtibial prosthesis would be most appropriate for which of the following individuals?

  a. An elderly man with a 15 degree knee flexion contracture and generalized osteo arthritis.

  b. A 30 year old public school teacher with a mature residual limb, who is 5ft 6 inches and weighs about 115 pounds. (x)

  c. A 20 year old Olympic heavyweight weight lifted with well developed muscular legs and residuum.

  d. A person who has been wearing a suction PTB prosthesis who is ready for a new limb.

CHECKOUT

- Which of the following criteria would in and of itself would make a unilateral transfemoral amputee NOT a candidate for prosthetic fitting?
  - a. A hip flexion contracture of 20 degrees
  - b. Grade IV cardiovascular disease (x)
  - c. A history of poor vision
  - d. Residual limb muscle strength in the Fair to Good range

- Which of the the following statements is *not* an indication for using suction to suspend a transfemoral prosthesis?
  - a. There is a scarred residual limb. (x)
  - b. The clients weight is stable.
  - c. The client has good balance.
  - d. There is a muscular residual limb.

- Initial prosthetic checkout is best performed:
  - a. after the client has completed gait training.
  - b. with an unfinished prosthesis on the alignment instrument. (x)
  - c. with the final finished prosthesis and new shoes.
  - d. whenever the prosthetist is available.

- Which of the following *is* a reason for aligning any above knee socket in some adduction?
  - a. To allow the amputee to sit more comfortably
  - b To reduce pressure on the greater trochanter
  - c. To allow for contraction of the tensor fascia latae
  - d. To improve mediolateral stability on stance (x)

- While performing an initial checkout for a transtibial prosthesis, you ask the client to walk a bit in the parallel bars. When you remove the prosthesis to check the

residual limb, you notice that there are sock marks over the distal end of the residual limb and proximally to above the gastrocnemial bulge. There are no marks over the crest of the tibia. There are no sores or abrasions on the residual limb. Which of the following is correct?
a. the socket is too tight proximally.
b. the stump sock marks are in the proper place. (x)
c. there is no distal end total contact.
d. the suspension cuff is too tight.

- For optimal gait pattern and good stability, it is desirable to align the transfemoral prosthesis so that the residual limb is held in:
a. full extension and neutral abduction.
b. slight flexion and slight abduction.
c. slight flexion and slight adduction. (x)
d. full extension and slight adduction.

- A client walking with a transtibial prosthesis that is too long will most likely exhibit which of the following gait deviations?
a. Ipsilateral pelvic rise on prosthetic stance with lateral trunk bending (x)
b. Contralateral pelvic rise on prosthetic swing with lateral trunk bending
c. Contralateral knee extension with lateral trunk bending
d. Ipsilateral knee flexion greater than 15 degrees on prosthetic stance with no trunk bending

- When doing a checkout on a client wearing a PTB prosthesis with cuff suspension, you can determine whether or not there is pistoning by:

   a.   drawing a line on the sock at the socket brim and watching to see if the brim drops on swing. (x)

   b.   observing the anterior brim of the socket to see if there is a gap between stump and socket on stance.

   c.   checking the stump after the client walks to see if there is redness over the midpatella tendon.

   d.   looking to see if the prosthetic toe is clearing the floor during prosthetic swing.

- A client with a 6-inch right transtibial residual limb was fitted with a PTB prosthesis with supracondylar cuff and SACH foot. Immediately prior to prosthetic fitting, the muscle strength in the right lower extremity was in the good plus range and the range of motion of the right knee was 135 degrees to 5 degrees. You are now doing the initial checkout of the PTB prosthesis on the alignment instrument and you note that the socket is aligned in 8 degrees of flexion. Which of the following statements is correct?

   a.   The socket needs to be flexed 15 degrees.

   b.   The socket should not be flexed.

   c.   The client should not have been fitted.

   d.   The prosthesis is properly aligned. (x)

- Six months later the same person appears, and you notice that he is wearing high-heeled cowboy boots. You recall that when you check him out he wore regular oxfords, and speculate about the effects the higher heels of the boots will have on his gait. You might see:

   a.   excessive lateral thrust.

   b.   foot slap.

   c.   premature knee flexion. (x)

   d.   pelvic drop in stance.

- Nancy Jones returns to clinic 1year after final checkout of her right PTB/SPSC prosthesis. On observation today you note that she is wearing one five-ply sock, her right hip drops a bit at midstance, and the distal end of the stump is a bit hard and callused. You check the pelvis and note that the right is one fourth of an inch lower than the left. The chart reveals that the pelvis was marked level on final checkout one year ago. Nancy has no complaints and there are no open areas on the stump. On the basis of the above information, you would conclude that:
  - a. the stump has probably shrunk and she is end bearing in the prosthesis. (x)
  - b. a one-quarter-inch difference in leg length is within normal limits and acceptable.
  - c. the checkout 1 year ago was inaccurate and the prosthesis is short.
  - d. she has probably changed shoes to one that has a lower heel.

- After you have determined whether or not Ms. Jones has a problem, what would you recommend?
  - a. A new socket
  - b. Adding a one-quarter-inch lift to her prosthetic shoe
  - c. Nothing, because her stump has no abrasion
  - d. Adding additional stump sock(s). (x)

- The PTB socket must be designed to give relief over which of the following structures?
  - a. The flares of the tibia
  - b. The shaft of the fibula
  - c. The head of the fibula (x)
  - d. The posterior soft tissues

- A client wearing a PTB prosthesis may have excessive distal end pressure on weight bearing if:

  there is too_____flexion in the socket.
  a. much
  b. little (x)

  the socket is too_____.
  a. tight
  b. loose (x)

  the client is wearing too_____ socks.
  a. few (x)
  b. many

- A client wearing a PTS prosthesis is found to have an excessively wide base gait (greater than 5 centimeters). Which of the following is *unlikely* to be the cause?
  a.   A medial leaning pylon
  b.   Hip abductor pathology or weakness
  c.   An overlong prosthesis is too long
  d.   Excessive foot density (foor is too hard) (x)

- While checking the fit of Joe Paternack's newly fitted ischial containment socket, you notice that Joe is sitting on the mat table and is unable to reach down and touch his shoes. This indicates to you that:
  a.   the socket is too tight.
  b.   the pelvic band is too high.
  c.   the foot is improperly placed.
  d.   the anterior wall is too high. (x)

- Knee instability in the transfemoral prosthesis may be caused by:
  a.   a medial wall that is too high.
  b.   too much knee joint friction.

    c.   insufficient flexion of the posterior wall. (x)
    d.   insufficient adduction in lateral wall.

- A person walking with a transfemoral prosthesis that is too long may exhibit any of the following gait deviations *except:*
  a. lateral trunk bending over prosthesis.
  b. circumduction. (x)
  c. abducted gait.
  d. vaulting.

GAIT TRAINING

- Tommy Johns, a 19-year-old client fitted with an ischial containment socket and Seattle foot, is learning to go up and down steps without the handrail. Which of the following techniques would you teach him?
  a.   Lead with the sound leg, then push up on the toe of the sound leg and hike the prosthetic leg up on the same step.
  b.   Lead with the sound leg, then flex the hip and knee of the prosthetic leg while pushing up on the toe on the sound leg to bring the prosthetic leg up to the next step.
  c.   Lead with the prosthetic leg and throw the body weight up by pushing vigorously with the sound leg and bringing it up to the same step.
  d   Lead with the sound leg, then slightly abduct the prosthesis and flex the hip to bring it to the same step. (x)

- For an individual with a transfemoral amputation, the best method for going up hills or ramps is:
  a.   leading with the prosthetic leg.

    b.   leading with the sound leg. (x)

    c.   leaning forward.

    d.   keeping the body weight on the prosthetic heel.

- Control of the prosthetic knee in gait is achieved by teaching the client to:

    a.   extend the residual limb against the posterior wall of the socket at heel strike. (x)

    b.   flex the residual limb against the anterior wall of the socket at toe off.

    c.   bend the trunk forward at heel strike to bring the CG anterior to the knee joint.

    d.   extend the trunk backward over the prosthesis at mid stance of gait.

- The best method for a person wearing a transfemoral prosthesis to climb stairs step over step, is to place the prosthesis on the step and then _____ and _____ the residual limb to pull his or her body up on the step.

    a.   extend, abduct

    b.   flex, adduct

    c.   extend, adduct (x)

    d.   flex, abduct

- An individual learning to walk with a PTB prosthesis, must learn to:

    a.   hike the hip on swing.

    b.   bend the trunk laterally over the prosthesis.

    c.   flex the knee slightly HS to midstance. (x)

    d.   extend the hip at heel strike.

- Which of the following statements concerning a client walking with a Canadian hip disarticulation prosthesis is *not* true?
  a. The pelvis on the amputated side will drop down on stance as the soft tissue is compacted.
  b. The client will have more difficulty with knee control than if walking with an AK prosthesis. (x)
  c. The client will take shorter steps than if walking with an transfemoral prosthesis.
  d. An elastic strap is used to decelerate the limb at the end of swing.

- Which of the following statements concerning individuals with bilateral amputations is *not* generally true?
  a. Individuals with two prostheses will tend to walk with a somewhat more widely based gait than unilateral amputees.
  b. A person with transtibial and transfemoral amputations is more likely to become a successful prosthetic wearer if he or she was initially a successful unilateral transfemoral prosthetic wearer.
  c. Functional outcomes of prosthetic training are directly related to the balance, strength, and coordination of the client as well as to the level of amputations.
  d. The elderly person fitted with two prostheses is generally best trained to walk with a walker for safety and stability. (x)

- You are teaching Ms Thomaston, the 78 year old mother of a close friend, how to walk with her PTB exoskeletal prosthesis suspended with the sleeve and fitted with the SACH foot. Ms Thomaston lives in San Francisco, a city of many hills, so she asks you the best method to go up the hill. You show her how to go up the hill sideways. Ms Thomaston, a curious lady, wants to know why she can't go up the hill step over step as she used to do. What would be the most accurate information to give her?

    a.   The prosthetic foot does not allow enough dorsiflexion to let her step through with the other leg. (x)

    b.   The socket is aligned in flexion, and it would hurt her residual limb to step through.

    c.   It takes too much energy to walk up a hill step over step.

    d.   The torque created by the extra contraction of the quadriceps could put her knee under stress.

- The ability of a client with a transfemoral amputation to walk safely with a prosthesis is dependent on the client's learning to:

    a.   control the prosthetic knee. (x)

    b.   walk in a rhythmic manner.

    c.   flex the prosthetic knee at terminal stance.

    d.   take even sized steps.

- A walker is not the ambulatory support of choice for someone with a unilateral lower limb amputation, because:

    a.   it forces the client to walk slowly.

    b.   it interferes with a normal gait pattern. (x)

    c.   it prevents the use of hands for ADL.

    d.   it is not covered by Medicare.

- A stretching sensation at the end of the transfemoral residual limb on weight bearing in the prosthetic socket indicates that the individual:
  a. is wearing too many socks. (x)
  b. is internally rotating the prosthesis on donning.
  c. has shrunk and is falling too far in the socket.
  d. has a neuroma on the incision line.

UPPER EXTREMITY PROSTHESES

- Which of the following is *not* a class of prosthetic hand?:
  a. Active-assisted (x)
  b. Passive
  c. Voluntary-opening
  d. Voluntary-closing

- The grip strength of a body-owered upper-xtremity terminal device is proportional to:
  a. the number of rubber bands around the hook. (x)
  b. the strength of the sound upper extremity.
  c. the amount of force exerted by the individual.
  d. the degree of tightness built into the terminal device.

- The above-elbow harness functions in all of the following *except:*

  a. transmission of power to flex the prosthetic forearm.
  b. humeral rotation control. (x)
  c. locking and unlocking the elbow unit.
  d. operating the terminal device.

- In general, the most important component of any upper extremity prosthesis is the:

  a. socket.
  b. terminal device. (x)
  c. suspension.
  d. elbow lock.

- Upper extremity prosthetic function is most limited by:

  a. lack of sensation (x)
  b. poor cosmesis
  c. sockets which are too hot
  d. loose suspension

THE CHILD WITH AN AMPUTATION

- Sally Smith, a 6-month-old infant with a left below-elbow transverse hemimelia and right congenital apodia (absence of a foot), has been referred for prosthetic recommendation. Assuming the child is developmentally normal, which of the following would be the best recommendation?
  a. Fit Sally now with a below-elbow banana socket with a passive mitt and plan to fit with a Symes prosthesis at around 9 to 12 months, or when she starts to pull to stand. (x)
  b. Fit Sally now with a powered below-elbow prosthesis with a functional plasticized hook and a Symes prosthesis.
  c. Fit Sally now with a Symes prosthesis and plan to fit with a myoelectric below-elbow system when she is about 12 months old.
  d. Recommend delaying any fitting until Sally is at least 1 year old and is better able to adapt to a prosthesis.

- Which of the following is *not necessary* to successful rehabilitation of a congenital upper extremity?
  a. Proper fitting of myoelectric prosthesis (x)
  b. Acceptance of the disability by the parents
  c. Integration of age related functional activities
  d. A supportive school environment

- Which of the following correctly states one reason disarticulation amputations are recommended in children, especially if amputation is through diaphysis?
  a. Bone overgrowth occurs most often in tibia and fibula.
  b. Soft tissue is not mature enough to provide adequate nourishment for the healing of a more distal amputation.
  c. Disarticulations are faster and less painful.
  d. Bone overgrowth occurs most often in the femur. (x)

- Slim Jim is a 6-month-old male who has a left terminal transverse hemimelia, above the elbow. As he grows, you would expect the residual bone to:
  a. grow longitudinally and circumferentially (x)
  b. grow only in the longitudinal direction.
  c. grow only in the circumferential direction.
  d. not grow at all due to lack of epipheses.

- The best time developmentally to fit a child with a congenital upper extremity amputation is
  1. when he or she begins to walk independently.
  2. when he or she begins to sit independently.
  3. when he or she begins to cruise.
  4   when he or she begins bilateral activities.

a. 2 and 4 (x)
b. 1 and 3
c. 2 and 3
d. 1 and 2